Staying ON I
Great Reset

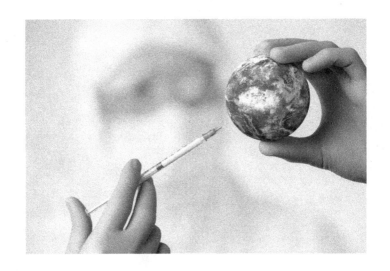

K. M. Patten

Staying ON During the Great Reset

Other books by K. M. Patten:

Indictments from the Convicted: Rants, Articles, Interviews and Essays

Staying ON During the Great Reset ©2022 K. M. Patten, All Rights Reserved

Print ISBN 978-1-949267-85-3
ebook ISBN 978-1-949267-86-0

This book is sold subject to the condition that it shall not, by way of trade or otherwise, be lent, resold, hired out or otherwise circulated without the publisher's prior consent in any form of binding or cover other than that in which it is published and without a similar condition including this condition being imposed on the subsequent purchaser.

Cover design by Guy Corp, www.GrafixCorp.com

STAIRWAY≡PRESS

STAIRWAY PRESS—APACHE JUNCTION

www.stairwaypress.com
1000 West Apache Trail, Suite 126
Apache Junction, AZ 85120 USA

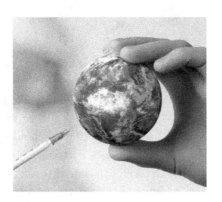

Staying ON During the Great Reset

Klaus "Mr. Reset" Schwab

THERE WERE A lot of dishonest people who cheered for the initial lockdowns of early Twenty-Twenty. Throughout all the state requirements and later "recommendations," the average Ze and Zir lockdowner had assured us that these measures were only temporary. We just had to hold our breath, wrap ourselves in some paper and plastic, warn our kids against killing someone, and then kick the rest of our loved ones far away from us.

Not much to ask for.

And then, eventually, one day—the exact date was deliberately left uncertain—we would reach the point of some mythical "reopening." *At last, the return to normal!* But few lockdowners are willing to admit that normalcy was never in the cards.

In fact, the explicit goal of global elitists like Klaus Schwab is the ushering in of a "New Normal." A protégé of Henry Kissinger, Schwab is the forebear of "stakeholder capitalism," which cannot be divorced from a certain kind of progressive activism. He's also the founder and director of the World Economic Forum, a global organization that works closely with the World Health Organization, and which advises leaders from around the world (Davos, anyone?), including one Joe Biden.

Schwab and co-author Thierry Malleret were kind enough to draw a framework for this…yes, agenda, there in a book-sized essay available on Amazon. They wrote it right smack in the middle of Year One, June 2020, with the title as an announcement: *COVID-19: The Great Reset*. "People feel the time for reinvention has come," Schwab writes cheerfully.

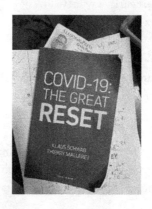

Staying ON During the Great Reset

So epochal is this moment in time, that Schwab (from here out, I'm just going to quote the book solely as Schwab's, since his co-author seems to be a comparative nobody), citing nobody, says that "some pundits" refer to the years before 2020 as "BC," with the years thereafter as "AC." "COVID," as one would guess, replaces Christ as the "C." (No, blasphemy is not an item discussed in the book.)

While admitting that the current pandemic should not be given a "superficial" analogy with historical plagues like the Black Death, Schwab does believe that it's caused more "human suffering and economic destruction" than the 2003 SARS outbreak, as well as the 2008 financial crash. Then he wonders if it'll be worse than the 1918-1919 Spanish Flu.[1] (That's what they're now saying).

And he's honest enough to admit that the harms of "the pandemic" entail more than just the deaths caused by the virus, as he talks candidly of the increases in the cases of domestic violence and psychiatric illness following the initial lockdowns.

Schwab's obsession for this project gets tiresome, with words like "necessary" and "urgently" hammered repeatedly into the text. "We'll never get back to normal," he writes declaratively. But why this pandemic? Won't it eventually pass like all the others?

For Schwab, that doesn't matter, because we're living in a time that is ripe for permanent change, this due to technological advancements and the growing acceptance of globalism, and we must now take "advantage of this unprecedented opportunity to reimagine our world, in a bid to make it a better and more resilient one as it emerges on the other side of the crisis."

First, the world's population—and by that Schwab means their respective governments, whom he loves—must work together to not only end the current pandemic, but to prevent any future pandemics from getting out of hand. Decrying the rise of nationalism and what looks to him to be a "global order deficit," Schwab writes:

> *This will only come about through improved global governance—the most "natural" and effective mitigating factor against the protectionist tendencies. However, we do not yet know how its framework will evolve in the foreseeable future. At the moment, the signs are ominous that it is not going in the right direction. There is no time to waste. If we do not improve the functioning and legitimacy of our global institutions, the world will soon become unmanageable and very dangerous. There cannot be a lasting recovery without a strategic framework of governance.*

Secondly: the advancements in technology have presented the opportunity in which to implement what is sometimes referred to as a "biosecurity state." In short, this means mass surveillance, with Schwab making sure to feign concern about privacy. Still, we'll soon have "many animated conversations" about the "trade-off" between individual freedom and "public-health benefits." One would expect a pushback against these intrusions.

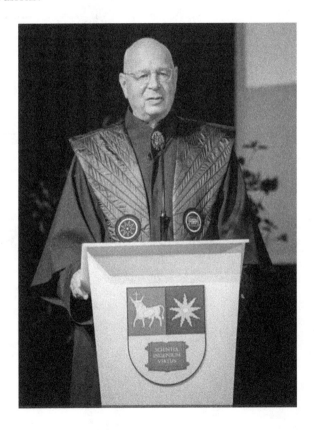

Thankfully, according to Schwab (who again forgets to offer any citation), the populations in the U.S. and Europe are all in favor of giving governments the authority to track smartphones. Go democracy! "The containment of the coronavirus pandemic," Mr. Reset writes ominously, "will necessitate a global surveillance network capable of identifying new outbreaks as soon as they arrive." There on the page, you can practically see the blushing on Mr. Reset's face as he writes about the possibility of tracking an individual's movements in "real time," with the ultimate purpose of enforcing a lockdown with more procession.

Staying ON During the Great Reset

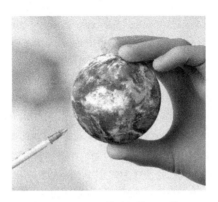

The Resetted Ideologues

BUT NONE OF this can happen without some help, and so what Mr. Reset needed is the assistance of Ze and Zir lockdowner.

Anyone seeing oppression in clothing[2] and arithmetic is going to wish for their own kind of "reset," and now they're helped along by wealthy and powerful men (sometimes European, oftentimes not, rarely women) whose whole objective is to create a new epoch with the aid of supra-technologies.

Perhaps it's only a coincidence that your neighborly mandator mainly comes from the Left side of the spectrum, but, all the same, Mr. Reset gives thanks by making sure to check-off all the usual progressive boxes: global warming, wealth inequality, gender and racial oppression, etc. (LGBTQ and BLM are spelled out specifically).

"There is little doubt," he says, saluting and thanking the tragically Resetted, "that it will be the catalyst for change and a source of critical momentum for the Great Reset." By "it," Schwab means two things: the social activism of the younger generation, and the activism found in "stakeholder capitalism."

The theory, from my understanding, entails pretty much anyone who is in any way connected to an entity that has been incorporated: customers, employees, suppliers, and all such broader communities. Needless note: governments invest in a great deal of industry, and so their input is an easy given. "Companies," writes Schwab, "will not necessarily adhere to these measures because they are genuinely 'good,' but rather because the 'price' of not doing so will be too high in terms of the wrath of activists, both activist investors and social activists."

These idealists share with Mr. Reset the goal of changing society, and they start with the elimination of consistency, both morally and intellectually. For example, those who rage endlessly about right-wing fascism had nevertheless argued that it was not a "lockdown," but instead a "public safety measure."

Yesterday we were told to respect someone's ownership of their own body, and today we'll learn how we're all medi-collectivized due to our potential to kill someone with a cough or a handshake.

Then scratch your head as I do: exactly how are we supposed to enforce all these draconian policies after the nation's police forces have been properly defanged? (a test of loyalty and a correction of principles: how many U.S. police officers actually have arrested Americans that defied the lockdown?)

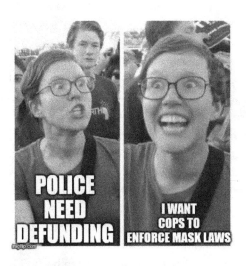

Meanwhile, any unspent energy will be directed, not towards the consideration of opposing arguments, but towards the destruction of capitalism—but only so long as massive information-controlling corporations obey their friends in the federal government and thus censor those who say things they have no courage to hear.[3]

Hoping not to get dizzy, one can then see the Lockdown Lefties applauding the decisions made by property owners who conduct business and offer employment, but only when it involves the possibility of checking someone's vaccination status; or, for more ideological backflips, the rightwing willingness to use the state to tell both Big Tech and all smaller businesses what they're allowed to do and not do. (Although, to be fair, I don't know of many Republicans who believe that businesses should have the right to discriminate based on other categories, such as sex, race, religion, or disability).

The reset is disappearing logic itself! Schwab's minions imagine a world in which inconstancy is a virtue, and not some sort of error or pragmatic approach.

How have the people tolerated, for almost two years now, this flicking of the reset button? If we were truly headed for a technocratic dystopia, wouldn't there have been some kind of civil war before then? Not necessarily (and it could still be on its way). For every society has suffered its own unique madness, and within those national madhouses has existed a sizeable part of the population that harbors fantasies of rising above the stained ceilings as they make their way to becoming one of the despots. Everyone else who doesn't want those people hanged calls them "brothers and sisters," or "my fellow countryman." With that, there's either a rabid desire to see violence, or a stronger hesitancy for seeing it through; all the while, the ropes that hold together any remaining national unity continue to rot and come undone. Through those windows, one can see democracy—at least federal democracy—for what it actually looks like.

Luckily for the aspiring Stalins of our own generation, they have now been given the most perfect opportunity in which to oppress: the deadly virus of 2020 definitely does kill, it often seriously injures, it's at least as communicable as the flu, and therefore let's stop everyone on earth from taking one step further until the virus has evaporated with the cough of the last infected person. The crisis, as imagined, ends boringly with a snotty tissue, not claiming a single life more.

This strategy makes sense, for a second.

But it's not the effects of the virus that makes the lockdowners foam at the mouth. Rather, it's finding out their neighbor has realized the full scope of the consequences. That is: if people are not allowed to make a living, forbidden from visiting friends and family, and hindered in our efforts to take proper exercise, then the corpses that inevitably show up elsewhere will be given longer descriptions on their death certificates.

Yet the networks stayed committed to ignoring the ugliness of insolvency, to say nothing of mental and physical decay. Nearly two years into the pandemic, and we can now see the results, intended or not.

For instance, those in U.S. who worry about emergency rooms being inundated with COVID cases should be made aware that those hospitals also cared for a huge influx[4] of young women who had attempted suicide, a 26% increase since all this started. This is on top of a 31% increase of all teenagers who went to the ER because of a mental health related incident, as well as a record number[5] of drug overdoses.

How few testimonies have been heard about these

sufferers, or those who have lost savings, or those whose businesses went under. Or the countless more who've missed the comfort of company and the outdoors. At best, these scenarios lead—have led—to drug addiction and suicide and financial ruin. At worst, a funeral that nobody will be allowed to attend.

The gravediggers on MSNBC and CNN are aware that headlines of "overdose and suicide" don't activate the response systems quite as urgently as "death by highly-contagious coronavirus," which is the main reason why they refuse to give any real coverage to those casualties. *You can kill yourself, beat up your wife, sleep in the street, or gain 50 unhealthy pounds—just don't infect me, because I'm getting paid handsomely for pushing this Great Reset thing.*

The propagandists have turned on the projector full-speed and put it right next to our heads. If the bat virus hasn't by now burrowed into your lungs, it has surely sunk into your consciousness. We can't think of anything else except its lethality. Now, the question of its origins is one that daily evades us. Don't speak of old antivirals as possible treatments. Say nothing about probiotics, or melatonin, or monoclonal therapies. Exercise and fresh air? *How bizarre.*

Instead, hyperfocus on what the virus does; after all, you might've personally seen it kill and maim, and in the strangest and most random patterns ever witnessed. Why not help it become *the* medical mystery of the 21 century? This will surely inflate the panic, the thing that's needed in order to distract from a reality that is constantly getting turned off and on with every shrill voice that comes out from a colorful glass screen.

Suddenly, the average Joe and Jane American begin to think that the paranoia of Ze and Zir lockdowner was not without merit. They then start feeding off one another's selfishness, rarely wondering about anyone else, and losing any mind for something as silly as *medical freedom* or *alternative treatment*. Neither seem bothered at the ease in which a powerful state might soon offer the choice between getting a vaccine (more on the Vaccine soon) and enjoying public life.

In short, the reset agenda has willing participants, both on the street level and the higher levels. And while it might be silly and *superficial* to call this a religion, plenty of Great Resetters borrow a method from the soon-foregone monotheisms, that by using violence and hypocrisy as axes in which to climb to the top of a promised holy land.

For our discussion, the Mask Question demonstrates perfectly the problem of blind faith coupled with unyielding obedience. Why, no matter how much evidence there is pointing to the inefficacy of widespread masking (do read the lengthy review of mask studies at AIER[6]), do the Resetters insist that everyone should be made to wear one? This includes children, who are hardly affected at all by this virus.

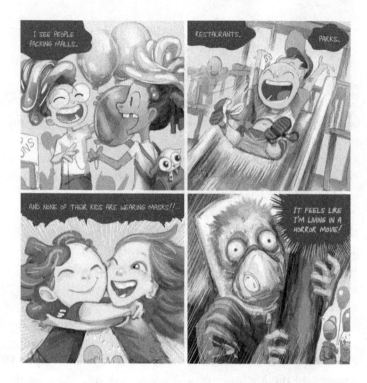

The CDC finally got around to studying the question in late 2020. For this, they took a close look at the Georgia school system, covering 169 schools in the state and more than 90,000 elementary students. This was the largest study yet conducted in the U.S. on the virus-slowing protocols we've all taken part in.

In May of 2021, the CDC published their results. While

they found there to be some benefit of masking teachers and providing better ventilation to the classrooms, the masking of children did "not have a statistically significant benefit," writes David Zweig for *New York Magazine*.[7] This part of the study seems to have been omitted from the online summary, and then ignored by everyone except the "fact checkers," who have been hard at work shouting about the "missing context."

Did the CDC then reverse its position based on new evidence? Of course not. *Time to Reset!* Until recently, item Two on their official website read: "Due to the circulating and highly contagious Delta variant, CDC recommends universal indoor masking by all students (age 2 and older), staff, teachers, and visitors to K-12 schools, regardless of vaccination status."

Ze and Zir lockdowner were likewise unpersuaded, and so continue to regurgitate the narrative sprayed at them by the cartoonish people on the screen. Both dismiss the notion that children should be able to tell the difference between smiling, grimacing, or sulking, and that the voices and words around them should be heard as clearly as possible. Unlike the mandators in the media, safely held in place with no mask in sight, your neighborhood mandator usually has to repeat themselves several times, as their own piece of fabric saves us from having to entertain such callous stupidity.

Or perhaps the agenda goes further than we think. Maybe pop victimization has found new venues in which to make noise. After all, resetters are really amused at the sight of children handicapped in their efforts to get a restorative intake of our invisible life force. Do these same people also laugh at friends who attempt to covey emotion without the full impact of facial expressions? One can almost envision the soon-to-be headlines: "Your child needs to check their oxygen privilege"— "the racist origins of using your lungs"— "You don't suffer mental illness as bad as I do because I don't even move my face when I talk."

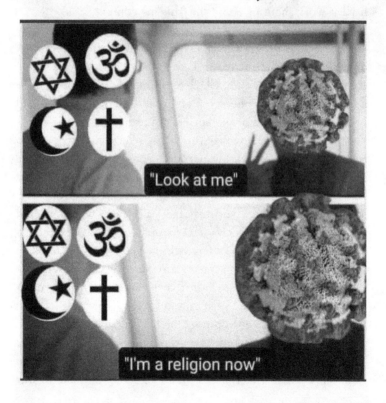

Staying ON During the Great Reset

This train of thought reminds me of some of the discussions I've had with "believers in Christ." There's an exhaustive aftereffect without the reward of any mind getting changed, which is a process much different than being "resetted." It's for good reason, I think, that the term "Branch Covidian" has found its way into our language, as the religious/cult-like element is hard to understate.

Absolutists burn, bury, or eschew contrary evidence as a matter of principle, but at least Schwab acknowledges the horrors of the lockdowns, as well as attempting to debunk the "façade" of individual liberty (that's the word he used).

The main drivers, the ones making this New Normalcy accepted, are a mob of people who are just as boring as Schwab, but with one more honest than the other. Who knows: maybe they'll one day take after their benefactor and start wearing cool Reset vests. That'll put an end to the comparison with faith, definitely.

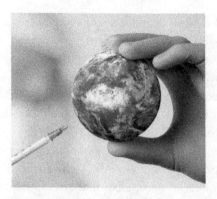

Scandals, Immunity, and the Vaccine

IF ONE WERE conspiracy-minded, one might assume that a technocratic elite were hoping, if not planning, for the outbreak of a very lethal virus. In the high-tech 21st century, total containment of such a virus would surely give rise to an authority so large and so monolithic that no freedom would fail to find itself underneath its shadow. "Governments," says our globalist savior, "must do and spend whatever it costs in the interests of our health and our collective *wealth* for the economy to recover sustainably."

This would be a globalized state that's powerful enough to initiate a lockdown at a second's notice, with always enough fiat currency conjured up as needed. Schwab's desired society is one in which you, the average citizen, receives routine notifications on your smartphone, all of them sent by some sort of Global Pandemic Command Center. The messages will inform when the most recent lockdown has been lifted, following the quarantine of a dozen or so infected neighbors. You would then be permitted to go outside and get your groceries. And then, looking like some faceless, hunched-over figure, you can take those pieces of paper to an Essential Store, with all involved bodies remembering not to stand too closely together.

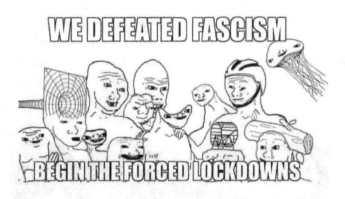

Yet even that won't get you in the door. *The Vaccine!* Schwab's manifesto—written in the middle of 2020, when Operation Warp Speed was in full swing—has eight references (by my count) regarding the incoming chemical. One reference serves as both the promised panacea as well as a self-contradiction: "[A] full return to 'normal' cannot be envisaged before a vaccine is available." But I thought we were never returning to normal?

In our current situation, not yet arrived at Schwab's

utopia, there's hardly a headline that's absent the "V" word, and they're often accompanied with news about fresh mandates and the firing and quitting of employees that refuse to get it. Each one of us, we're told, has a responsibility to receive the new vaccine, because once we've all been jabbed, the pandemic will be over. The amount of times this flimsy theory has been asserted only rivals the number of booster shots given to Ze and Zir lockdowner.

Until then, those who remain unvaccinated are not much different than mass shooters, their spittle akin to bullets being sprayed into a helpless crowd. Even scarier: there seems to be millions of these murderers (perhaps billions, if counting those globally), every one of them guilty of spreading disease and causing death. Your neighbor, therefore, should be presumed as pathogenic—a possible killer of you and your family.

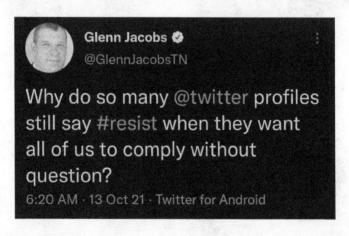

Such rhetoric has reached a fever pitch, and to spare your sanity, don't dare scroll on Twitter. As President Biden said, when asked about Facebook allowing "anti-vax" information on their platform: "They're killing people...really." [8]

This line looks to have hooked quite a few, including activist giant and pioneering scholar Noam Chomsky. "I have the right not to get vaccinated," Chomsky moralized in a recent interview, "but I don't have the right to run around harming people." He is far from alone in this kind of thinking. "It is your right to refuse to get a vaccine, but then it is your responsibility to isolate yourself, so you don't harm others," Chomsky stated while picking up his establishment credentials.

Which brings us to the first of several ongoing scandals.

A quick Google search will yield several articles regarding the inaccuracy of the COVID tests.

Examples are as follows.

At the beginning of the year, in January (2021), the FDA alerted patients and health care providers about the risk of false positives from the "Curative SARS-Cov-2 test."

The test was later pulled.[9]

Then, in the middle of the year, a team from the University of California in San Francisco studied 14 different tests used to measure antibodies in people who had been infected. "All of these people definitely had COVID, but not all of them had COVID-19 blood tests," reports Reuters.[10]

Finally, just this last November (again, 2021), the Australian company Ellume identified two million home tests that were giving exceedingly high "false positives," according to VeryWellHealth. This resulted in a Class 1 recall, the most serious type of recall.[11]

These stories are in addition to much talk that the PCR test—the "gold standard" for testing—has a lot of its own problems.[12]

The next question is obvious: How then are we supposed to know how many people have actually recovered from the virus?

A headline from the October 29th 2020 issue of *The Wall Street Journal* gives the answer: "No One Knows."[13] One can only guess the amount of people, throughout the world, who were once sick with the novel virus, but who never got tested with the novel metrics.

Even if it were possible to find out, the answer could spoil the plans of those trying to push universal vaccination. One can then see the full scope of this scandal, for it seems that no government, technocrat, or Resetter wants to acknowledge the reality of *natural immunity*.

Maybe they might not want to know how effective it is at stopping further spread.

That's not just conspiracy-mongering.

Robert Kennedy Jr.'s Children's Health Defense was curious as to how many people with natural immunity had been reinfected before giving it to someone else. They then filed a Freedom of Information Act with the Center for Disease Control (CDC) requesting their data on this subject. The agency responded by revealing that it does not collect such data.[14]

I do not pretend to be the first to make these points. Indeed, some Republican senators are trying to pass legislation that would formally recognize the protection conferred from disease recovery. (The Brownstone Institute—started by well-known libertarian Jeffrey Tucker as an effort to mobilize new, emerging, free institutions to replace the old, oppressive, and failed institutions—has been reporting on this area of study.)[15]

To those who wish to trust their own antibodies, the Center for Disease Control gave an unsurprising response: get the vaccine anyway. They've even created a new name for their experiment: "hybrid immunity." As it is, the CDC likely spends more money on the invention of terminology rather than the study of vaccines.

Now we come to the real scandal—the vaccine itself. One will have probably heard that this vaccine isn't a "real vaccine," because, unlike all other vaccines, this one contains no trace particles of the actual virus at hand (this includes the vaccines made by Johnson and Johnson and AstraZeneca, which uses a "modified" vector virus)

The two other main vaccines being used, produced by Pfizer and Moderna, use the mRNA technology. The technology itself has been getting worked on for around thirty years, with early hopes to be used against cancer, but this is the first time it's been rolled out, here in the big leagues of COVID.

For this subject, who better to talk to than the man who made the main contribution to its development? This happens to be the same scientist who's been sounding the alarm as to the vaccine's potential harms. On his Twitter bio, Dr. Robert Malone deems himself the "inventor of mRNA vaccines and RNA as a drug." Some outlets have tried to debunk Malone's claim, insisting that the vaccine is here only through the work of many different scientists.

As far as I can tell, that's both true and untrue, and best left to personal interpretation. Dr. Malone was kind enough to talk to me on the phone, that for about 45 minutes. "Did you read the article in *The Atlantic*?" he asked me. I said I had. He considered it a hit piece, and with a title like "The Vaccine Scientist Spreading Vaccine Misinformation," one can see why.

Still, the article cites a lengthy history of the work done on "messenger RNA," conducted for Ghent University in Belgium. Malone's scientific research, done at the Salk Institute (San Diego, CA), are the first two citations out of 224. The paper's lead author, Rein Verbeke, told *The Atlantic* that Malone and his co-authors "sparked for the first time the hope that mRNA could have potential as a new drug class."

But this essay is not intended as an exhaustive history of the vaccine's development, nor to question Dr. Malone's contribution to it. Dr. Malone's time during those early years was traumatic, and as such, he did not feel like discussing that period at any length. (To make up your own mind, I urge readers to follow up with at least two other documents: a massive 7,000-word article[16] written by his wife, Jill, as well as another history published by *Nature*, entitled The Tangled

History of mRNA Vaccines.[17] Both are listed in the references at the end).

Even if the vaccine was a collaborative effort, no source I've come across ever attempts to deny the man's game-changing contribution.

And yet, Malone says that he's the "most vilified scientist on the globe," adding plainly that he's "suppressed." Is he not? Aside from an interview with Tucker Carlson, Malone isn't found anywhere in the "legacy media"; that is, on one of the major network conglomerates.

His suppression should be seen as yet another scandal.

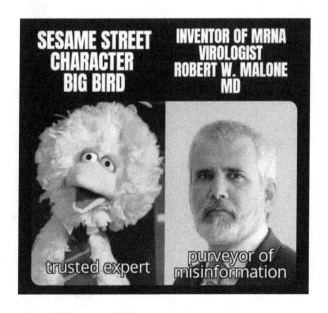

In June of '21, Malone appeared on a podcast with Bret Weinstein and Steve Kirsch. For more than three hours, the three men discussed their concerns about the vaccine. "I became concerned earlier than the [podcast], but not much earlier," he tells me. Malone originally got a phone call from a CIA officer who was in Wuhan, China, where the outbreak first started. "He said I better get my team ready, because it looks like it might be a bad one," Malone says.

A Canadian immunologist named Byram Bridle had gotten ahold of the "common technical document" (information about the medicine) for the Pfizer vaccine. It was then passed along to Malone, who was asked by Trial Site News to give a review.

Malone tells me:

> *I found that there were enormous shortcuts taken in the nonclinical testing prior to the initiative of the clinical trials. I was quite shocked by what I saw. They were basically allowed to cobble together data that was obtained for other purposes and was not specific to the vaccine, which had not been done rigorously, and then submit that to the regulatory agencies worldwide in support.*

Malone, who has managed projects worth eight billion dollars in grant money, says he found it "personally offensive," because the "norms of my industry that I'm trained in and had to live with for thirty years were just completely disregarded." Citing the estimated twenty thousand deaths reported to the VAERS system (the Vaccine Adverse Event Reporting System), I then asked him what damage, he believed, the vaccine had already wrought. "Direct causation," says Malone, restating the common complaint, "is really impossible to establish with VAERS system. But if you use standard methods for correcting for the under-reportage, methods that were developed 10-20 years ago, it looks like the VAERS reports are about forty-fold underreported."

VAERS is a "no fault" system, meaning that if a plaintiff does manage to prove that a vaccine has caused injury, the semi-secretive court can award financial compensation. But here's the difference: when any other product—say, a vehicle, treadmill, or a baby's crib – is found to have been the cause of death or injury, a judge will rule that the *manufacturer* is legally at fault. As the gavel goes down, the words "you are responsible" are put into the record.

These words are not, and cannot, be spoken at the vaccine court. This is because the 1986 legislation that created the court (signed hesitatively by President Reagan) grants indemnification to the pharmaceutical companies for their production of vaccines. With this most insidious logic, it can always be stated that compensation did not prove causation. Vaccine manufacturers need not do anything more: neither to recall their product, redesign the formula, nor even issue stronger warnings. Thus, business carries on undeterred.

As for the adverse effects of this vaccine, Dr. Malone tells me that "myocarditis is one that the CDC officially recognizes." This was a matter of "signal to noise ratio, the ability to detect statistically." Because myocarditis and pericarditis (inflammation of the middle layer of the heart wall, and inflammation of the tissue around the heart, respectively) are so rare amongst children, the signal is easy to pick up.

Malone elaborates:

> *The signal was originally detected by a group at the FDA, that I've interacted with for years, that was working with one of the senior biostatisticians from the company Oracle, who brought some advanced statistical techniques for assessing clinical data, that automatically corrected for what's called 'confounding,' which is this problem of when there's a background level of some event and then you're having an increase from an intervention. The FDA, which uses really antiquated methods, to match their antiquated database, hoped they could rely on the Israel database to detect rare adverse events. But the Israelis had not detected myocarditis and pericarditis. So this group that was outside of the review branch, outside of the vaccines division, at the FDA, together with this Oracle biostatistician,*

> *did detect that signal, then alerted both the CDC and the Israelis, and the Israelis then verified that they could detect the signal once it had been identified. Then once they could confirm the signal was there, the CDC confirmed they could detect the signal. This took two months.*

Malone says he already knew this was the "main adverse effect," as did his colleagues. And like the vaccine itself, that associated side effect is constantly making new headlines. Expectedly, most of these seek to downplay the risk. Worse, one soon reaches a kind of "infobesity": one study says one thing ("hardly any risk at all"), another study says something different ("cases are mild and easily treatable"); back and forth, until you're so overwhelmed with the contradictions that you forego the formation of an opinion. However, as Malone pointed out to me, some European countries have halted the use of Moderna's vaccine for men under the age of 30. That should speak to something.

But here's the undeniable nub: *they've lied about the vaccine in another way*. Who is "they"? I asked Malone at whose feet would he lay down the blame. "Fauci," he answered. Of the man Malone has met several times, he says: "He's functionally in control of the entire NIH enterprise as it relates to these vaccines." What Fauci and the Resetters have lied about has already been mentioned above. A video on BitChute, entitled "They Lied About the Vaccine," [18] offers a compilation of high-profile persons stating that the vaccine will stop the spread of the virus, only to later admit that—well, no—it actually does not.

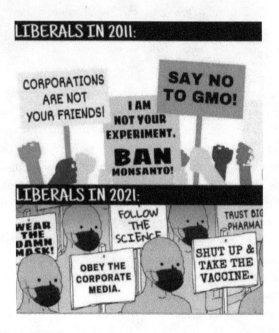

Roll tape! (All of them stated in 2021): The President of the United States, Joe Biden: "You're OK, you're not gonna get COVID if you have these vaccinations." (July) CDC director Rochelle Walensky: "Our data from the CDC today suggest that vaccinated people do not carry the virus." (March) Bill Gates on baseless conspiracies: "Will it hurt the vaccine uptake, where everyone who takes the vaccine is not just protecting themselves but reducing their transmission to other people and allowing society to get back to normal?" (January) Fauci: "It's such an important imperative of why those regions, those people, need to get vaccinated: to protect themselves, to protect their community, to protect their family." (June)

A couple months later, and it's already time for a reset! Biden: "Earlier today, our medical experts announced a plan for booster shots to every fully-vaccinated American…eight months after you've got your second shot." (August) Walensky: "What they can't do anymore is prevent transmission." (August) Gates: "We got vaccines that help with your health, but only slightly reduce transmission. We need a new way of doing vaccines." (November) Fauci: "When you look at the level of virus in the nasopharynx of people who are vaccinated, who get breakthrough infections, it's really quite high and equivalent to the level of virus in the nasopharynx of unvaccinated people who get infected." (August)

As far as I'm concerned, this is a checkmate. Any rebuttal given by the Resetters will only serve as a concession to the basic argument put forth by us skeptics, which is that the vaccine has not been studied long-term, and therefore we would hold off. But for the Resetters, that's unacceptable. The human race will always be obligated to get the jab, lest civilization come to an end.

Did the theory go implicitly as such: the vaccine is rolled out in December of 2020, and then the following month, all eight billion people on the planet would be vaccinated, thereby destroying the virus once and for all? That scenario, of course, is insane. There weren't that many doses; children were not yet approved; and there was always going to be vaccine refusers. Finally, Fauci himself had originally said that herd immunity, via vaccine, was not a short-term plan.

If making up the science was an Olympic sport:

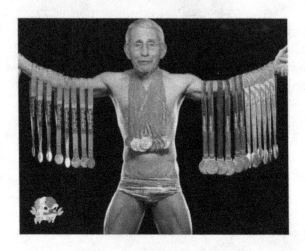

But as everyone knows by now, Fauci changes his position about as often as he does his tie. Soon later, he said that even deadlier variants could appear if we don't get everyone vaccinated. After that, he said that the vaccine worked well against the variants (Also, some scientists, including Malone, think the variants are coming about because of mass vaccination).

It's almost as if Tony "I am the science" Fauci is making this stuff up as the months go on.

At best, the man is a charlatan; at worst, he's a psychopath. A true scientist with integrity would have told the public: this is the first time the mRNA technology has been used, and we're not sure exactly what to expect. Then conduct some clinical trials, make it entirely voluntary, and allow free individuals to decide for themselves.

Why didn't Fauci, or anyone else, state this? To sell a vaccine? To usher in The Great Reset? What scandal were we on?

On these matters, the reader can make up their own minds. Nevertheless, starting from mid-2020, right up until Summer of 2021, we were told that things would return to normal once the vaccine hit the market.

That didn't happen, despite many populations having high rates of jabbing.

As I pointed out earlier, some elites never intended for a return to normalcy. While The Great Reset agenda carries forth, the rate of "breakthrough cases"—the vaccinated contracting the virus—continues to skyrocket. "We have a suboptimal leaky vaccine that isn't preventing spread very well," Malone says, which is why you have to "get the jab again and again and again."

Even during the holiday season of 2021, Fauci instructs[19] us all to get vaccinated so as to *stop transmission of the virus* ("If you want to keep the level of spread as low as possible, which will get us back to that level of normality, you have to get those people vaccinated")

Yet, at the same time (in December), Fauci signs his name onto a commentary published by The *New England Journal of Medicine* which states: "Vaccination has also been unable to prevent 'breakthrough' infections, allowing subsequent transmission to other people…" [20]

Amid the pandemic, DoubleSpeak has been on grand display. A Resetter can say one thing, and then almost immediately contradict themselves, with hardly two breathes in between.

If one scrolls through social media, or visits their favorite lefty city, they'll likely find people who still insist vaccination as the way to "stop the spread."

As to why that is, Malone tells me: "We have a population that has been subjected to a psychological operations campaign."

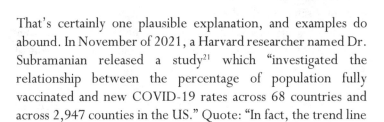

That's certainly one plausible explanation, and examples do abound. In November of 2021, a Harvard researcher named Dr. Subramanian released a study[21] which "investigated the relationship between the percentage of population fully vaccinated and new COVID-19 rates across 68 countries and across 2,947 counties in the US." Quote: "In fact, the trend line suggests a marginally positive association such that countries with higher percentage of fully vaccinated have higher COVID-19 cases per one million people." To give a summary is to repeat what's been said above, which is that the vaccine is ineffective, and may even be causing the virus to spread further.

This study proved popular among the vaccine's critics, those who Malone says are "vilified" and "slandered" and "professionally attacked." Perhaps that's why the author of the study quickly went on record to say his work had been misrepresented. What we should take away from the study, Subramanian said, is that we need to do more—you guessed it—hand-washing, mask-wearing, and social-distancing. Any other suggestions—say, focus on early treatment—might have cost him his job.

As can be seen, those who are pushing this agenda have pledged their allegiance to a new faith. There are few pushing the vaccine now who had asked way back then: What if this vaccine doesn't work the way they said it would? And if the initial statements about the vaccine's efficacy turned out to be untrue, is it possible that the current statements about the vaccine's safety might also prove to be untrue?

During my talk with Dr. Malone, he wondered whether he would ever be compared to Oppenhiemer, who of course created the atom bomb. After reciting Oppenhiemer's famous quote about Vishnu— "I am become death"—Malone warns: "I'm not saying I'm as brilliant as Oppenheimer, nor that the mRNA vaccines are as deadly as thermonuclear weapons, although time might show otherwise." And if they lied about this vaccine, what's to say they won't lie about the next generation of mRNA vaccines?

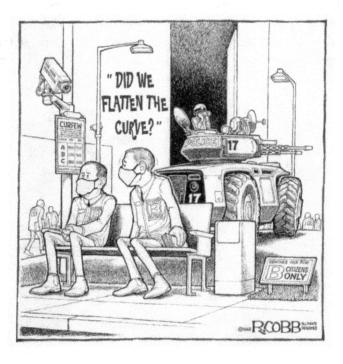

Reset resisters, and Ze and Zir lockdowner, Joe and Jane American, and citizens around the world, all need to decide where they're at on the chessboard, and what move they hope to make next. Schwab and his World Economic Forum are hard at work trying to set up a global vaccine passport system. At the same time, there's already talk of a fourth booster shot. They're also coming for our children, who are hardly affected at all by the virus. It's "obscene," Malone says on that last point. "The data are quite clear that the risk benefit ratio is upside down for children." For we who resist medical fascism, I have a few suggestions as to how we can take control of the Reset Button.

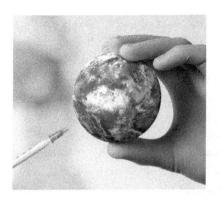

Taking Control of the Reset Button

EVEN WITHOUT SCHWAB'S godlike aspirations, the world is still undergoing radical changes. Advancements in technology, new means for acquiring knowledge, and ethics that must bound to evolve, would all seem to demonstrate this. Though global elites dream of taking control of these shifts and powers, their authority has yet to be shown as legitimate. There's no reason why they should have the final say in how the future is shaped.

So where do we go from here? What steps should be taken to resist the Reset, successfully stop medical fascism, and perhaps even create a better tomorrow for ourselves and our children?

Our first step, I think, is to recognize how bad the situation is getting. At the start of 2022, twenty-two states in America have passed mandate legislation.[22] Because of the U. S. Supreme Court ruling, these mandates are allowed for workers in healthcare. As for the corporate world, information is still coming in. One survey[23] of large U.S. employers found that one-quarter of them were going ahead with vaccine mandates, with or without the Supreme Court's approval. Just turn on the news, and chances are you'll soon hear about the latest mandate. Worst of all, a recent Rasmussen poll showed that many Democratic voters support federal vaccine mandates, as well as locking down those who refuse to get jabbed.[24]

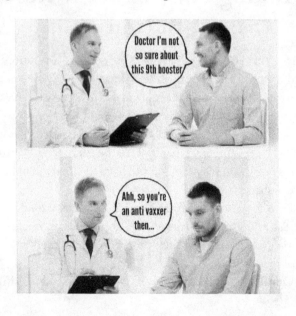

Staying ON During the Great Reset

The second step in stopping this tyrannical trend is to draw lines in the sand. As hard as it might be to do, those battle-lines must be made. It's important to be aware of who around you perceive your life as meaningless should you not go along with the Reset. As I pointed out in Section Two, Lockdown Lefties care about oppression only insofar as they can do some of it themselves. They enjoy gaslighting we who resist by arguing that none of these measures amount to "real oppression." These are the types who supposedly care so much about the working class, but when they hear about workers being laid off for refusing the jab, they quickly recall their primary objective—the end of white supremacy! —and then promptly dismiss their plight.

Often, they do this by deploying the cheapest form of "WhatAboutism," asking smugly: "What's the matter? Don't you remember slavery, or Jim Crow? Doesn't feel too good, does it?" (I'm thinking of bigoted lefty hatemongers like Tim Wise, who wrote an article[25] that essentially said the same thing, although those are not direct quotes).

Because these bottom-feeders suffer from vengeance-induced myopia, it does not occur to them that people of color are also negatively affected by mandates and lockdowns. But as long as white workers also feel some pain, it's all the better.

Even though the dishonesty of Ze and Zir lockdowner knows no limits, it's still fairly easy to realize when you're in the midst of an enemy. Indeed, medical mandates coming from the state *are* oppression.

Don't ever let these rabid fascists tell you otherwise.

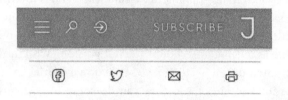

You Know Who Else Opposed Vaccine Mandates? Hitler.

BY
BRANKO MARCETIC

Contrary to claims about "fascist" vaccine mandates currently circulating on the Right, the Nazis actually *relaxed* German vaccine mandates — and hoped doing the same for

And while we're drawing these lines, we can also be forging new coalitions. Individuals and groups that you would have before been feuding with might now be potential allies. For instance, I am neither a conservative, a Christian, or a Republican. If I had to make use of labels, I'd consider myself a secular libertarian (albeit one that might be seen as leaning to the right), as well as a student of the original anarchist, William Godwin. As a Godwinian, I'm very much in favor of progress (the eventual perfection of mankind!), which would prohibit me from "conserving" every single thing done in the past. And as a secularist, I am opposed to theism and absolutism, of which I have opposed all my life, with no expectation of that changing.

However, most of those who stand opposed to these mandates come from the right side of the aisle. For the sake of both freedom and the future, I'd be willing to put aside my other critiques and work with Christian Conservatives towards that singular goal. After all, Reset theism is closer to being legislated into my life than Christian fundamentalism.

But there's a few things I'd like to point out to my new allies. For one thing, while plenty of Christians have been opposing the Reset, many others are helping it along. An Associated Press article from September 2021 was titled: "Many Faith Leaders Say No to Endorsing Vaccine Exemptions." [26] The piece lists the heads of various denominations who have excoriated those wishing to receive a religious exemption. These include: the Christian leaders of the Greek Orthodox Archdiocese of America, the Evangelical Lutheran Church in America, the Roman Catholic Archdiocese of New York, and the U.S. Conference of Catholic Bishops. To name a few. How ironic to find Christians helping to bring about the Mark of the Beast! Then I ask: What side is your congregation on? And where does your own allegiance lie? Implore! Draw those lines!

Police are another concern. I've yet to find a comprehensive study or report that attempts to tally up the number of Americans that were punished in 2020 merely for defying the lockdown orders. But there were many—sunset-watchers, churchgoers, and countless business owners—all of whom received fines and/or put in cuffs. We await that total. And who made that possible? The same ones who find their support base amongst Christian Conservatives. For this, we find insight from the great Thoreau. In his classic 1849 essay, "Civil Disobedience," [27] Thoreau explored ways in which righteous individuals could oppose an unrighteous state. His metaphor for those state servants is useful here:

> *The mass of men serve the state thus, not as men mainly, but as machines, with their bodies. They are the standing army, and the militia, jailers, constables, posse comitatus. In most cases there is no free exercise whatever of the judgement or of the moral sense; but they put themselves on a level with wood and earth and stone; and wooden men can perhaps be manufactured that will serve the purpose as well. Such command no more respect than men of straw or a lump of dirt. They have the same sort of worth only as horses and dogs.*

And so! The Resetters have dreams of domination, but they

rarely have nightmares of their enforcers abandoning their posts. They fully expect there to be an army of men and women made from wood and stone who are content to trade brutality for a paycheck. Battling their own cognitive dissonance, Christian Conservatives will excuse and defend the police by saying that they're "just following orders." This reaction is laughable, especially since they'll soon remind us how soldiers in the Third Reich had done the very same thing. Coming forward, they'll then applaud the protestations of those who work in hospitals and airlines. Police, somehow, are exempt from this moral standard.

Thoreau was not so understanding. For the state enforcers plagued with guilt, he had a solution: *resign!* Dig your soul out from underneath the inorganic material and tell your superiors that you will no longer be the vanguard for high-tech fascism. They may take your pension, but your conscience will remain intact. Or, should we tell citizens of other western democracies that they should "back the blue," even as the "blue" is beating them down for their defiance?

To stop the Reset, there must be a mass of resisters. And all resisters ought to be imbued with a constitution that might require a certain amount of personal sacrifice, of individuals willing to say no—despite the worse that can happen.

Losing a job or pension is an easy and fairly painless example. Here's a tougher one: There's been several (conservative) critics of medical fascism who've contracted the virus only to later die from it. Whenever that happens,

Resetters have themselves a hearty round of schadenfreude. But even in light of those deaths, we must be willing advance the causes of liberty, bodily autonomy, and parental jurisdiction.

In other words, even if COVID-19 were to kill me tomorrow, I still would not want my child to grow up into a world in which he'll be forced to inject experimental chemicals into his body. I might be hooked up on a ventilator, with tubes and wires sticking out of my pallid body, and yet the thought I would dread most would not be of my heartrate flatlining, but rather the prospect of my child being told to receive his annual booster.

Because regardless, the risk for all such injections rests entirely with us, with none given to the companies that make them, and hardly any for the tyrants that push them.

As Robert F. Kennedy Jr. has reminded everyone, the Founders of this country believed there were worse things than death. "We have to love our freedom more than we fear a virus," Kennedy says.

The Resetters stand no chance if confronted with a mass of men and women who have made that same determination.

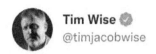

Tim Wise ✓
@timjacobwise

Parents getting mask/vax exemptions from chiropractors or pastors (?) should get a visit from Child Protective Services. If your kid has a real condition that might qualify for an exemption get your PCP to sign off on it. Otherwise, you're a shit parent who needs a case opened

2:50 PM · Sep 16, 2021 · Twitter Web App

32 Retweets **2** Quote Tweets **198** Likes

Of course, we don't wish for death or maiming by the virus, which brings us to our next step. It has been known, and for a long time, that obesity is a major cofactor for complications from COVID-19. Be shocked and horrified to learn that America is far and away the most obese nation on the planet! As for children, an article from TheConversation.com [28]lists a number of studies showing how the majority of kids hospitalized with COVID complications were—and are—either overweight or diabetic. "A large study of more than 43,000 hospital presentations of children under 18 years old in the United States showed the main background health conditions that increased the chance a child would need admission to hospital with COVID were diabetes and obesity," the article states.

To echo an oft-made observation, if the authorities had truly cared about health, then the playgrounds and parks and gyms would have remained open rather than the liquor stores. But they didn't care, and we can now see the consequences of their actions, as another study shows that children got a lot fatter during the pandemic.[29]

We resist now only the urge to be conspiracy-minded, as maybe the bastards desired a new generation of overweight, unhealthy humans. Then we can see something that is completely within our hands, a step to be made and followed by many more, until a few of us have shed a few pounds and thus reduced our risk of a severe outcome should we contract the virus. This includes our children, who should never be forbidden exercise, fresh air, and sunlight. (On that last one, there's growing evidence that vitamin D—which we get naturally from the sun—reduces one's chances of severe COVID complications.)

On the most personal level, optimizing our health and having therapeutic protocols in place are things we can all do, either individually or within our families and communities.

Staying ON During the Great Reset

What about the political and social levels? As for the former, people living in civil society will inevitably wish to use the state apparatus to preserve their liberties. As an anarchist, this method irks me; yet even I can recognize the utility of it. Whether by vote or by decree, Resetters are already harnessing the power of the state. Why shouldn't we also attempt the same? I won't argue that the effort is unwise. I'd only argue that it should not be our first mode of resistance. Thoreau said voting was:

> *A sort of gaming, like checkers or backgammon, with a slight moral tinge to it, a playing with right and wrong, with moral questions; and betting naturally accompanies it. The character of the voters is not staked. I cast my vote, perchance, as I think right; but I am not vitally concerned that that right should prevail. I am willing to leave it to the majority.*

A lot of advocates for medical freedom insist that we cast our vote for Republican candidates. And, as said earlier, while a lot of Republicans are opposed to vaccine mandates, how many Republicans, in 2020, had gone along with the lockdowns? Nearly all. So what if a Republican gets into office, perhaps even the Highest Office, and then appoints a disciple of Faucism, thereby enacting another nationwide lockdown? How would we know that such a candidate hadn't recently attended one of Schwab's summits? Should we then take notice of all the conservative activists who vote for a Republican only to later decry them as a RINO? Finally, could we find ourselves staring out of a window, watching federal police patrol our streets, while wishing we had heeded Thoreau's gambling metaphor?

Dismissing my pointed questions, Republican poll workers will chide us, saying how we are responsible for the Reset lest we march down to the polling booth and mark that "R." But I think we've all experienced enough gaslighting in these last couple years; there's no reason to endure any more of it, especially from people who agree on the basic principles. None of this is to say that we should never vote for a Republican; it is only to warn against betting all of our chips on one candidate. And even if we did elect a Republican, that politician's feet should never rise higher than a few inches above the proverbial fire.

Besides, there could be a more practical way to get involved with the political process, one that doesn't require undying allegiance to either of the two corrupt parties. As far as I am aware (although check your state rules, because the rules are probably different state-by-state), one need not be a Republican or a Democrat in order to introduce a measure onto a ballot. Ballot referendums could be used to enshrine the principles of liberty, at least within the twenty-six states that allow for them (for the twenty-four that don't, perhaps those voters should change that).

Staying ON During the Great Reset

What would we, a resisting electorate, wish to pose to the rest of our fellow voters? A measure could read something like: "No agent of the government will ever have the right nor the power to restrict legal public activity—yes or no?" A majority who marks "Yes" will have hopefully restrained any official, present or future, from ever again enacting another lockdown, with the threat of hard punishment always hanging above them.

But what if they vote "no"? Let's explore the issue a little further, because, while the federal state should not have the power to enact lockdowns or to forcibly inject chemicals into your body, both individual states and private businesses are a different matter. Here, pure libertarians will find themselves conflicted. If a business is sovereign, should they not be allowed to set their own rules? If a business wants to mandate vaccines for their employees or customers, that's their right. Isn't it? Well, my hope would be that a vigilant public would use their purchasing power to bankrupt any business that attempted mandates. Of course, so far, things aren't looking that way, with the majority of workforces getting jabbed, whether happily or grudgingly.

Then should we pass a law or ballot measure prohibiting businesses from enacting mandates? Constitutionally, it's very much a double-edged sword. The debate about "federal verses state power" has been raging since the beginning of our country, and as such, it could go either way. Thomas Jefferson, primary author of the Declaration of Independence and the Bill of Rights, as well as the third President of the United States, believed that the individual states had even the power to shut down newspapers. If that were so, then the states could make such prohibitions. But then they might even have the right to enact more mandates and lockdowns.

Admittingly, there's no easy solution for this. Personally, I could tolerate a society that had a few small businesses that catered to people who wanted to associate only with others who are vaccinated. But then, I'd also prefer to live in a society in which the whole population was educated enough to realize that the vaccine *doesn't stop transmission!* This is where we can take the next step: to be the ones who do the educating! One can already see how easy it is to strike up conversations about vaccine mandates, medical fascism, and the overreach of the state. It often happens almost at random, and no state or corporation could ever stop us from talking to other like-minded freedom fighters. Neither could they stop us from attending protests and rallies and making our voices heard. These are great, practical, and easy ways to resist the Reset.

These spontaneous conversations could serve as the catalyst for the emergence of new institutions, and indeed a more enlightened populace. Imagine the possibilities! That collective energy could give birth to a world in which men like Schwab, Fauci, or Biden are never given any kind of power or influence. Or one in which corrupt medical establishments like the CDC were replaced by ones that actually listened to their patients, and treated them as individuals. Or one in which propaganda outfits, like the legacy media, or "comedy shows" like Saturday Night Live, would only be seen in the archives of a library. Or one in which Big Tech was made obsolete, because we all found ways to keep in contact and organize without the need for their platforms (imagine never again seeing someone's pronouns in their bio). Or one in which school unions started adhering to the will of the parents, and not the other way around.

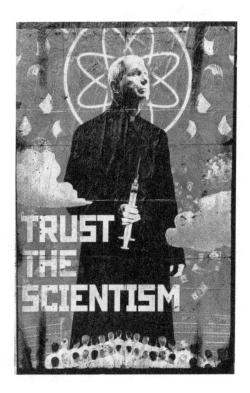

If Schwab can have his dreams, then so can I. And so can you. Schwab envisions a future in which the world has made a successful "green recovery." Ostensibly, this is essence of "Build Back Better." And while renewable energy is a respectable goal that can be shared by anyone, there is something frightening about the prospect when it's advanced by men who state that: "Dystopian scenarios are not a fatality," assuring us that "the genie of tech surveillance will not be put back into the bottle." Behind the philanthropic, feel-good talk about a world in which robots do the bulk of the labor, while we sit comfortably entranced in our simulated metaverses, there is sinister and authoritarian intent. I myself am all in favor of seeing a better world; and yes, one that realizes renewable forms of energy. And I'd hope that such a future was presided over by human beings who are less dogmatic, less violent, and more concerning of people besides themselves.

We don't need Schwab, Biden, or any medical fascist to help us achieve those goals. The only cost of this New Normal would be a society made to accept lockdowns at random, personal activity constantly monitored, and vaccines no one could refuse. Don't expect any such measure to be given so much as a proper public debate.

As for our current situation, don't get too hopeful about the recent Supreme Court ruling shutting down President Biden's federal mandate. Although many states, cities and businesses are now rescinding their own mandates, the Resetters are likely regrouping to try again. I think they will find as many variants as needed in order to make their dream—our nightmare—a reality.

With that, there's no time to lose, and we must all start resisting.

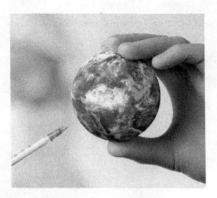

End Notes

[1] https://www.smithsonianmag.com/smart-news/the-covid-19-pandemic-is-considered-the-deadliest-in-american-history-as-death-toll-surpasses-1918-estimates-180978748/

[2] https://www.yahoo.com/now/did-bernie-sanders-inauguration-outfit-epitomize-white-privilege-a-san-francisco-teacher-thinks-so-204425621.html

[3] https://www.yahoo.com/now/biden-raises-fears-big-tech-193200466.html

[4] https://www.usnews.com/news/health-news/articles/2021-06-11/big-rise-in-suicide-attempts-by-us-teen-girls-during-pandemic

[5] https://www.commonwealthfund.org/blog/2021/drug-overdose-toll-2020-and-near-term-actions-addressing-it

[6] https://www.aier.org/article/masking-a-careful-review-of-the-evidence/

[7] https://nymag.com/intelligencer/2021/08/the-science-of-masking-kids-at-school-remains-uncertain.html
[8] https://www.nytimes.com/2021/07/16/us/politics/biden-facebook-social-media-covid.html
[9] https://www.fda.gov/medical-devices/safety-communications/risk-false-results-curative-sars-cov-2-test-covid-19-fda-safety-communication
[10] https://www.reuters.com/article/health-coronavirus-science/covid-science-antibody-test-reliability-faulted-new-predictor-of-covid-19-severity-idUSL1N2P628Z
[11] https://www.verywellhealth.com/ellume-recall-covid-home-test-fda-5209140
[12] https://www.rcreader.com/commentary/questioning-unreliable-pcr-testing-is-hardly-trivial
[13] https://www.wsj.com/articles/how-many-have-recovered-from-covid-19-cases-no-one-knows-11603963801
[14] https://childrenshealthdefense.org/defender/cdc-data-natural-immunity-covid/
[15] https://brownstone.org/articles/79-research-studies-affirm-naturally-acquired-immunity-to-covid-19-documented-linked-and-quoted/
[16]
https://static1.squarespace.com/static/550b0ac4e4b0c16cdea1b084/t/60b62e4f1dcb1f52ad2d4c0c/1622552143483/Jill%27s+letter+about+RNA+vaccination+generic+v5+June2021.pdf
[17] https://www.nature.com/articles/d41586-021-02483-w
[18] https://www.bitchute.com/video/f20b9dAcqJku/
[19] https://www.cbsnews.com/news/fauci-covid-omicron-variant-herd-immunity-vaccine-infection/

[20] https://www.nejm.org/doi/full/10.1056/NEJMp2118468
[21] https://pubmed.ncbi.nlm.nih.gov/34591202/
[22] https://leadingage.org/workforce/vaccine-mandates-state-who-who-isnt-and-how
[23] https://www.shrm.org/resourcesandtools/hr-topics/benefits/pages/despite-mandate-many-employers-move-toward-requiring-covid-vaccines.aspx
[24] https://www.rasmussenreports.com/public_content/politics/partner_surveys/jan_2022/covid_19_democratic_voters_support_harsh_measures_against_unvaccinated
[25] https://goodmenproject.com/featured-content/covid-anti-vaxxers-are-the-ultimate-snowflakes/
[26] https://apnews.com/article/health-religion-united-states-coronavirus-pandemic-coronavirus-vaccine-9c947acecd6ba26b4c78827b7b87c185
[27] https://www.gutenberg.org/files/71/71-h/71-h.htm
[28] https://theconversation.com/it-might-be-uncomfortable-to-talk-about-but-obesity-puts-children-at-risk-of-severe-covid-171116
[29] https://www.cdc.gov/mmwr/volumes/70/wr/mm7037a3.htm

CPSIA information can be obtained
at www.ICGtesting.com
Printed in the USA
LVHW091320220322
713984LV00023B/712